qualified physician. The intent of this book is to describe my personal experience regarding my heart disease. If medical advice or other expert help is needed, the services of an appropriate medical professional should be sought.

Chapter 1

I owned my individual Chiropractic practice, about 2 miles from my house. On February 28, 2001, as I was getting in my car to go home after work, I felt a severe, sharp pain in the left side of my chest. I was taught that the symptoms of a heart attack that men generally felt was like an elephant sitting on my chest and/or a tingling in my left fingers and left hand. I did not have the symptoms of a heart attack and did not know what was happening to me. After I drove home, I asked my wife to drive me to the Emergency Room. Since I had chest pains, I was admitted immediately and an electrocardiogram was taken. I have no family history of heart disease.

Before I continue with my story, let me say that I learned a lot more than I really wanted to know about my heart and the nature of my disease, congestive heart failure. I will review the structure of the heart and congestive heart failure. The heart is composed of special muscle cells that readily transmit electrical (nerve) signals. The heart is broken up into 4 chambers, the smaller upper 2 chambers, the atriums, and the 2 larger lower chambers, the ventricles. Deoxygenated blood flows into the right atrium. The blood then flows through a heart valve, the tricuspid, into the right ventricle. The tricuspid valve keeps blood from flowing back into the right atrium. Blood then flows through the right ventricle into the lungs, where it is re-oxygenated and then flows into the left atrium. Oxygen rich blood then flows through the mitral valve to the left ventricle and then the oxygen enriched blood flows out through the aortic valve to the rest of the body.

Congestive heart failure occurs when the heart cannot keep up with the body's demand for blood. This reduces blood flow to other tissues and causes blood to back up into the lungs. The blood flow from the left ventricle is measured by the amount of blood that flows (called the ejection fraction) to the body on each heart beat. Normally, the left ventricle pumps between 50 and 70 percent each heart beat. Congestive heart failure begins after the ejection fraction drops below 50 percent. Severe congestive heart failure occurs when the ejection fraction drops below 30 percent.

The electrocardiogram indicated that I had an irregular heart beat and a left bundle block of HIS (I could not find a definition of HIS, but it is also known as the atrioventricular bundle), the heart's natural pacemaker and the electrical conduction system of the heart. What this means is that the nerves attached to the left atrium and left ventricle were not functioning. Since the nerves from the right bundle were working, it took additional time for the heart muscle cells to conduct electricity to the left side of my heart and this put my heart out of rhythm, (arrhythmia).

I laid on a gurney in the ER for roughly eight hours until the blood tests indicated that my B Type Natriuretic peptides was in normal ranges and that I had not suffered a heart attack (myocardial infarction). B Type Natriuretic peptides is a measurement of muscle cell breakdown and is normally under 125 picograms per milligram for people under the age of 74 years and 450 pg/ml for patients, aged 75 through 99 years of age. I guess if you live more than 100 years you are out of luck. LOL! For patients under the age of 50 years, higher than 450 pg/ml is indicative of congestive heart failure and for people 50 years or older, higher than 900 pg/ml is indicative of congestive heart failure.

I was then scheduled for an echocardiogram to test the ejection fraction of my left ventricle.

I had a blood test on March 1 and a follow up exam with my primary care physician on March 5.

On March 8, I was given an echocardiogram to test the efficiency of my left ventricle and I was told that my ejection fraction, which should have been 50 to 70 percent was under 30 percent. An echocardiogram is a diagnostic ultrasound of the heart.

On March 16, I was scheduled for a Mugga Scan, where a mild radioactive substance was injected into my body and I lay under a scanning machine that recorded the radiation from my heart onto film. This is commonly called a nuclear study.

On May 8, I had an office visit where I was informed   that my ejection fraction was 21%. The test also indicated that I had had a prior infarction in the territory of the PDA (patent ductus arteriosus), (PDA is an abnormal blood flow that occurs between two of the major arteries connected to the heart; an infarction is the obstruction of the blood supply to an organ or region of tissue causing tissue death, thus myocardial infarction or heart attack results in necrosis, or tissue death in the heart muscle). The test also indicated that I was suffering from cardiomegaly, enlargement of the heart). I was given an estimate of less than 5 years to live.

On June 7, I was given a prescription for a beta blocker, which is used to manage cardiac arrhythmias and to prevent another heart attack.

Chapter 2

Now I want to describe my feelings and bit of my prior medical history. I had no family history of heart disease and the etiology (cause) was listed as unknown. My Chiropractic practice had gone from 5 days, 8 A.M. until 7 P.M., Monday through Friday, to 3 P.M. until 6 P.M. on Monday, Tuesday, Wednesday and Friday, a total of 12 hours per week. I did not have the energy to work any longer, but I still maintained a significant income. I thought my fatigue was caused by my age and sleep apnea. On January 20, 1998, I was diagnosed with severe sleep apnea and prescribed a CPAP machine to help me breathe while I was asleep. I kept falling asleep at my desk, but did not get the test until I fell asleep at a red light and was pulled over by police officer. He told me to go home and get some rest.

Over the next several years, my weight had been increasing because my activity level had greatly diminished. I began walking at night, but that was getting increasingly difficult to do. After I attended to my patients, I would fall asleep at my desk. When my office closed, my staff would leave for the evening and lock the front door. I would collapse in my chair and doze for 30 or 40 minutes and then drive the roughly 2 miles to my residence.

After dinner, I would usually doze off while watching television with my family. We had two children, a boy and a younger girl.

I would then stay up until after midnight and then go to bed. I was usually up by 9 or 10 A.M. I would sometimes have lunch with my wife, who worked at a local school district.

After I was informed that I had less than five years to live, I, at first, did not believe that was possible. I was stuck in this phase of grief for several years.

Over the next several years, I had a series of Encounters regarding my heart.

One the next page I will list the dates of the significant encounters, Emergency Room visits, etc. Blood tests, routine office visits, telephone appointments, etc. will not be listed unless they contain pertinent information. I was accused of being noncompliant by my Congestive Heart Failure nurse due to the alternative health care approach I was using to supplement my normal treatments. I saw this nurse practitioner on many of my routine office visits.

My symptoms included abdominal extension, bloating, angina (pains in the left side of my chest), shortness of breath, dyspnea (extreme shortness of breath upon exertion, orthopnea (shortness of breath while lying flat on my back), productive cough and weight gain.

One of the things I want to stress is how time consuming heart disease is. Suffering from a chronic disease such a congestive heart failure is also very expensive in the expenditures for travel, drugs and office visits and Emergency Room co-pays. From the time I was diagnosed with severe congestive heart failure, I had hundreds of encounters that included office visits, telephone consultations, blood tests, EKG's and echocardiograms

I have included my significant encounters with my heart to provide the time, effort and expense associated with my heart disease. Beginning in 2005, my HMO, Kaiser Permanente, began documenting all of their encounters on a computer. Prior to that time, I had copies of the hand written medical records recorded to a CD. I have read through 6,435 pages of medical records, with several hundred pages of handwritten notes. I was told that the handwritten notes may be incomplete.

February 25, 2006

An echocardiogram indicated that my ejection   fraction was 21% with a perfusion defect, moderate ventricular enlargement, mild tricuspid and mitral valve regurgitation, walls: septal hypokinesis (hypokinesis means weakly contracting muscle and the septum is the muscular part of the heart that separates the right and left ventricles).

April 19, 2005

A treadmill test was performed (a test to determine how the heart handles stress).

October 3, 2007

Emergency Room visit. Symptoms were chest pain and extreme shortness of breath while trying to sleep.

October 24, 2007

Office visit. Symptoms were seeing spots in front of my eyes that was like a prodrome (initial symptoms) to a classical migraine headache. I did not have the headache, probably caused by an excessive dosage of ace inhibitor drugs taken for my heart. Ace inhibitors relax the blood vessels to reduce stress upon the heart.

November 1, 2007

An EKG (electrocardiogram) indicated that my heart continued to have a left bundle block of HIS.

July 23, 2008

I went to the Emergency Room with symptoms of severe shortness of breath.

September 9, 2008

I underwent a nuclear study that indicated that my ejection fraction was 18%.

April 27, 2010

A blood test indicated that my B Naturetic Peptide (BNP) was 248, normal is under 125. Above 125 signifies the death of heart muscle cells.

January 4, 2011

I went to the Emergency Room with symptoms of extreme shortness of breath that had lasted for 2 days, a productive cough with clear sputum, able to speak only 3 to 4 word sentences due to lack of breath, unable to sleep at night and unable to ambulate (walk) more than a few steps at a time. My skin pallor was pale.

January 6, 2011

I was discharged from the hospital.

February 22, 2011

I had a consultation with a surgeon to determine if I was a candidate for a pacemaker (a Bi V ICD pacemaker with cardio defibrillator, non-ischemic dilated cardiomyopathy with LBBB (that means that the pacemaker will deliver an electrical shock to my heart under certain circumstances). The surgeon determined that I was a candidate for the pacemaker.

March 22, 2011

An EKG (electrocardiogram) indicated that my left bundle branch block was still present.

March 28, 2011

A pacemaker was implanted in the left side of my chest, above my heart, at Kaiser Permanente's Santa Clara Hospital.

March 30, 2011

I was discharged from the hospital.

April 3, 2011

I had a telephone call with a doctor. My symptom was an extreme shortness of breath.

April 6, 2011

I went to the Emergency Room and was admitted to the hospital for 2 days with symptoms of shortness of breath and chest pains. My pacemaker was checked (AIC interrogation indicated that an RV lead was not operating at maximum output). I was sent back to the Santa Clara hospital in an ambulance and I underwent surgery (my pacemaker leads into my heart were not responding properly, probably due to necrosis (tissue death) in my heart where one of the wire leads was touching my heart).

April 11, 2011

An echocardiogram was performed upon me that indicated mildly thickened mitral valve leaflets with moderate regurgitation, tricuspid valve with moderate regurgitation (heart valve leaks), my left ventricle was severely increased in size, my systolic function severely reduced (the phase of the heartbeat when the heart muscle contracts and pumps blood from the chambers of the heart into the arteries that service the heart and body). My ejection fraction was less than 20%.

May 12, 2011

I went to the Emergency Room for a cardioversion (an electrical shock to the heart) to get me out of atrial fibrillation (afib, where the atriums are out of rhythm). The attempt was made using my pacemaker as the cardioversion device. The technician inadvertently depressed the wrong key on his laptop computer before I was anaesthetized and it shocked me so badly that I felt as if I had bounced off the table. The cardioversion failed and I remained in afib.

September 2, 2011

I went to the Emergency Room with symptoms of dizziness and extreme shortness of breath. When I say shortness of breath, that generally means with exertion. When I say difficulty breathing, I have difficulty breathing. My blood test indicated that my BNP was 1593 (normal is less than 125), so there was a significant loss of heart muscle tissue.

September 3, 2011

I was discharged from the hospital.

September 17, 2011

I went to the Emergency Room with symptoms of severe breathing problems and was admitted to the hospital.

September 24, 2011

I was discharged from the hospital.

September 30, 2011

I went to the Emergency Room with symptoms of a stroke. I was admitted to the hospital with symptoms of aphasia (inability to speak or make any sound), right side facial droop, afib, both grips equal but weak, facial asymmetry, loss of consciousness, tongue deviation to the left, nonverbal, 4/5 motor control on the right side, patchy atelectasis of the right upper lobe of my lung (partial collapse). My BNP was 1997 which indicated I was losing significant amounts of heart muscle tissue. My symptoms began in the late afternoon hours when one of my wife's associates at work called to speak to her. My wife had not arrived home from work, yet. I had extreme difficulty in articulating words to her. She called my daughter and told her something was wrong with my speech. My daughter and wife got home around the same time. My wife asked me what was happening to me and I could not make a sound. Finally, my daughter asked me I wanted to go to the Emergency Room. I nodded my head yes and when I got to the Emergency Room, I was diagnosed with a stroke. Later, a neurologist told me that the stroke was probably cause by my afib condition. I regained my ability to speak within a few days. Before I was released from the hospital, I was told that my ejection fraction had deteriorated to single digits and that I had less than a week to live. I was sent home with morphine, which I never used, and was put on hospice care. I was taking oxygen full time. My brother and sister flew to Sacramento to visit me and say goodbye, as did my close friends who lived in the Sacramento region. My prayers were mostly for my family, but I did have a personal prayer that I would die in my sleep, while having a pleasant dream, pain free, and awaken in Heaven. I was put on hospice care. A nurse would visit me every other day and take vitals. A retired nondenominational minister would visit me twice a week. We would speak for a few minutes and then pray together. God Bless this minister!

I graduated from hospice care 6 weeks later and was sent back to my cardiologist for care. An echocardiogram indicated that my ejection fraction had improved to under 20% with a perfusion defect (passage of fluid through the circulatory system), moderate ventricular enlargement, mild tricuspid and mitral valve hypokinesis (weak contractions in the muscle cells between my ventricles).

December 29, 2011

An echocardiogram indicated that my ejection fraction was still under 20% and that I was suffering from aortic valve regurgitation, with moderate to severe mitral valve hypertension (indicating high blood pressure in the lungs), a severely dilated left atrium and left ventricle, my right atrium was moderately enlarged and my right ventricle was enlarged.

January 5, 2012

I was diagnosed with dilated cardiomyopathy (the heart becomes enlarged and cannot pump blood efficiently. This decreased heart function can impact the lungs, the kidneys and other body systems).

January 7, 2012

I was transferred to the Heart Transplant Unit in the hospital in Santa Clara (adjacent to San Jose). I was pale, but not cyanotic (blue). My wife said that my pallor was gray and that she feared for my life. My BNP was 1148. I was admitted to the hospital and began ultra-filtration, which extracted more than 30 pounds of water from my blood in 15 days. My symptoms were extreme shortness of breath and fatigue. Cardioversion was successfully administered and brought me out of afib. I had glomerular filtration (a test to determine my kidney function) and a catheterization (a long thin tube called a catheter is inserted in an artery or vein in the neck, groin or arm and threaded through the blood vessels and into the heart to examine the heart and arteries. My catheter was threaded through my neck). After my hospital stay, I could walk the entire length of my house, around 50 feet. Before I was admitted to the hospital in Santa Clara, I could only walk a few steps at a time and I was restricted to using an electric wheelchair to move around my house.

March 8, 2012

My BNP was 349, indicating heart muscle tissue loss.

March 28, 2012

I had an office visit in Santa Clara where I was notified that my BNP had improved to 227.

May 23, 2012.

I had an office visit in Santa Clara where I was anesthetized and my pacemaker was checked by giving me 3 cardioversions.

June 29, 2012

I had a blood test that indicated that my BNP had improved to 105 (normal is under 125).

October 3, 2012

I had a blood test that indicated that my BNP was 121.

October 14, 2012

I had an office visit in Santa Clara to check on the status of my heart.

January 14, 2013

I had an office visit to Santa Clara to check on the status of my heart.

May 16, 2012

I had a routine office visit in Santa Clara and was admitted into the hospital for an extended stay due to symptoms of extreme shortness of breath and pain in the left side of my chest.

May 27, 2014

An echocardiogram indicated that my ejection fraction had improved to 25 to 30% from under 20%. My heart valve leaks had improved from moderate to severe to mild to moderate.

July 29, 2014

I had a pacemaker check.

August 29, 2014

I had an office visit in Santa Clara to check on the status of my heart.

September 5, 2014

I had a pacemaker check.

October 10, 2014

I had a pacemaker check. My pacemaker battery was losing its charge.

December 4, 2014

My pacemaker was replaced in the Roseville Hospital.

December 30, 2014

I had an office visit in Santa Clara to check the status of my heart.

March 5, 2015

I had an office visit in Santa Clara to check the status of my heart. An echocardiogram indicated that my ejection fraction had improved to 40 to 45% and my heart valve leaks were negligible.

June 10, 2015

I had an office visit in Santa Clara to check the status of my heart.

June to August, 2015

I underwent cardio rehabilitation in a rehab center near my home.

September 4, 2015

I had an office visit in Santa Clara where I started taking half of my normal dosage of Lisinopril (ACE inhibitor). My nephrologist (a doctor that specializes in kidney diseases) had stopped me from taking an ACE inhibitor due to my kidney disease (caused by my heart condition).

March 15, 2016

I had an office visit and echocardiogram in Santa Clara that indicated that my ejection fraction had improved to normal ranges of 55 to 60%, that my heart had returned to normal size and that my heart valve leaks were still negligible. I had accomplished this miracle of the restoration of my heart function and size. I graduated from the Heart Transplant Unit in Santa Clara and was transferred back to the Roseville hospital which was near my home. HOORAY!!!!.

In July, 2005, I closed my practice in California when the worker's compensation laws changed making it extremely difficult for me to treat worker compensation (work comp) patients. My practice consisted mostly of work comp patients. I bought a practice near Birmingham, Alabama in order to be near my Mother (who was in her 70's) and my Grandmother (who was in her 100's). My physical condition allowed for me to practice 4, 3 hour days in California. The practice I bought in Alabama required me to work 5, 8 hour days. I had to treat many more patients for the same income. I began to suffer from symptoms of my heart disease almost immediately and had to go to the Emergency Room, twice.

After consulting with my practice management consultant, I advertised my practice for sale on the internet. I immediately found several potential buyers. I sold my practice within the week and agreed to stay for up to 3 months to help transition the new Doctor into the practice. The last weekend before Thanksgiving, the doctor who had bought my practice allowed me to leave and I spent Thanksgiving with my Mother. My wife, who was still living and working in the Sacramento area, flew out on the next day and we drove back to California.

After I returned to California, to avoid boredom, I enrolled in classes at my local community college and studied music, art, humanities, economics and math courses. Besides my Doctor of Chiropractic degree, I have an Associate of Arts degree, a Bachelor of Science Degree and a Masters of Business Administration Degree. I have always enjoyed college and I really liked the competition with my fellow students to have the best grades in each class. My ejection fraction was still below 20 percent and I did not feel well most of the time. Within a few years, my heart condition no longer allowed me to attend classes and I spent my time mostly reading, surfing the internet and watching television.

I have never been a candidate for a heart transplant or any kind of surgery to assist me with weight loss. The weight limit on heart transplants is 250 pounds and I am considerably heavier than that. I suffer from morbid obesity. I was told that I could not undergo any major surgery without a significant risk of death.

Due to my tolerance level for these drugs, I take only ½ dosage of the major drugs prescribed for congestive heart failure; beta blockers (used for treating abnormal heart rhythms and high blood pressure) and ACE (Angiotensin-converting enzyme) inhibitors (used for relaxing the blood vessels for an easier flow of blood taking strain off the heart muscle).

Chapter 3

Now that my ejection fraction and heart size are within normal parameters, I go to the movies and dinner at restaurants most weekends with my family. I still have other physical challenges, but what person who is close to 70 years old doesn't have physical challenges.

I am thankful for each day I awaken. I will now reveal how I achieved this miracle and how, in my opinion, any person with a heart condition can lengthen and improve the quality of their lives by following my protocols.

When I was told that I had less than 5 years to live in 2001, I sought after an alternative health care system. What I found was Ayurvedic medicine, which is the oldest known healthcare system in the world and was written about in the

Hindu text 'Rig Veda' more than 6,000 years ago. Ayurvedic medicine has been practiced in India for more than 6,000 years to treat diseases and health conditions and continues to be practiced today.

Shortly after I was diagnosed with severe congestive heart failure in 2001, I searched the internet for alternative medicines. I found in Ayurvedic the herb, arjuna, which uses the ground up bark of the Arjuna Terminalasis tree as a herb for treating heart diseases.

I began taking 500 a milligram capsule per day shortly after my diagnosis. By 2005, I had increased the dosage to 1 gram (1,000 milligrams) per day.

After my stroke in the fall of 2011, I increased my dosage to 2 grams per day.

On April 15, 2014, I read an article on the internet
about an experiment Ayurvedic researchers had conducted on mice with severe congestive heart failure. They gave the mice mega-doses of arjuna. Half of the mice recovered from congestive heart failure and the other half improved dramatically.

I began taking 6 grams of arjuna per day and my echocardiogram, taken in late May, 2014, indicated that my ejection fraction had improved from under 20% to 25 to 30% and my heart valve leaks had improved to mild to moderate from moderate to severe.

I increased my dosage from 6 grams to 8 grams of arjuna per day in July, 2014. In August, 2014, I increased my dosage of arjuna to 10 grams per day.

My echocardiogram on March 15, 2016 indicated that I had achieved my recovery from severe congestive heart failure and a severely enlarged heart in under two years after I began mega-dosing arjuna.

Arjuna appears to refurbish and rebuild the heart muscle but not the nervous system of the heart. I still have a left bundle block and my pacemaker keeps my heart in rhythm.

Arjuna is available almost anywhere in capsule or pill form. What I did was order a pound of arjuna powder. I mixed 4 teaspoons of arjuna with yogurt each evening. One teaspoon of powder is approximately two and one half grams of arjuna. So, I mixed in 4 teaspoons of arjuna with yogurt, spooned it down quickly and chased it with a sip or two of fruit juice. The yogurt makes the arjuna more palatable, but it still has an unpleasant taste.

Currently, you can purchase a pound (16 ounces) of powder on the internet for around $20. Two pounds of arjuna lasts about one year. It is a lot less expensive than taking arjuna capsules, which can be quite expensive.

If you are a heart transplant patient or have transplanted heart valves, I would suggest that you do not take arjuna until research is done on the effects of arjuna on a transplanted heart and/or transplanted heart valves.

I firmly believe that mega-doses of arjuna will extend and improve the quality of life for any person suffering from heart disease, unless you have had a heart transplant, and I strongly encourage any person suffering from heart disease to start taking mega-doses of arjuna. I would start with one teaspoon of arjuna a day for a week (one teaspoon) and then add a teaspoon each week until you are taking 4 teaspoons, daily. If you choose to use capsules, they typically come as 500 milligram capsules, though I have encountered 700 milligram pills. You would need to take 5 capsules per day for a week and increase your dosage by 5 capsules a day per week until you are taking 20 capsules per day (10 grams).

Now I look forward to each day instead of wondering if I will awaken the next morning when I go to bed.

I was 68 years old (almost 69) when my echocardiogram indicated that I had recovered from congestive heart failure. I suffer from morbid obesity (around 400 pounds on a 5 foot 7 and one half inch frame). My cardiologists told me they had never heard of a person recovering from congestive heart failure as I have.

It took 15 years and I was told in 2011 that I had less than one week to live and sent home with morphine (which I never used).

My wife is taking a gram of arjuna per day to help her avoid developing heart disease.

I sincerely hope that every person with a heart condition tries my plan. Godspeed and the best of luck to all of you.

Associated with congestive heart failure is kidney disease. I was told in 2015, by my nephrologist kidney specialist), that my kidneys were failing and that my kidney function was down to 30 percent. He said that dialysis was administered when kidney functions was down to 15 percent mark, but in my case, since I was a heart patient, that he would start me on dialysis when my kidney function was down to 18 percent. A year later, my kidneys had stabilized, much to my nephrologist's surprise, and he told me my kidneys should be stable for the remainder of my life. My next publication will be on how I stabilized my kidneys.